Brown Skin and Breast Cancer

P. J. HARGROVE

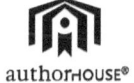

authorHOUSE®

AuthorHouse™
1663 Liberty Drive
Bloomington, IN 47403
www.authorhouse.com
Phone: 1-800-839-8640

This book is a work of non-fiction. Unless otherwise noted, the author and the publisher make no explicit guarantees as to the accuracy of the information contained in this book and in some cases, names of people and places have been altered to protect their privacy.

First published by AuthorHouse   12/28/2009

ISBN: 978-1-4490-6318-4 (e)
ISBN: 978-1-4490-6316-0 (sc)

Library of Congress Control Number: 2009913659

Printed in the United States of America
Bloomington, Indiana

This book is printed on acid-free paper.

This book is dedicated to women of all colors, who have or have had to deal with breast cancer.

And to;

Veda and Robin, I really feel that without you, I would not have made it through. Not in my right mind anyway. Thank you for being here. I'm glad that we are sisters and even happier that we are friends. You Rock!

Vicki, Diane, Gloria W. Gloria J. Linda B. Linda L. - to have one true friend is a blessing; to have you all in my life is a joy.

To the one woman who loved me, believed in me, and will always be with me, forever, you are on my mind and in my heart. Mom

In life we will struggle

Through ups and downs

But with faith, family and friends

We are never truly

Alone

Introduction

I wanted to start writing this so many times before. But I just couldn't seem to get it together and find a way to start. Each time I thought about trying, I talked myself out of it.

Who cares what you think? Who is really going to want to read this? Why do you think that anything you can say might make a difference?

Well, I finally decided to take that chance, because I just couldn't let go of something so important to me. I'm not even sure if anyone will be interested in what I have to say, but I just really felt compelled to share my story.

My hope is that some of you may find parts of this inspiring, helpful, and insightful. And yes, even a little humorous at times.

While I was going through this ordeal, it was very difficult for me to find information on how some of us were dealing with the changes that were going on. I don't know if it's because of where I live, or just that there wasn't much out there. If it was there, I couldn't find it. So I decided to try and change that. Not just for myself, writing has always been a type of therapy for me, but I really am hoping that someone will read this and know that what they've been through though lonely and extremely difficult, has really made them a stronger person. Maybe something that I say will make a difference for you.

I'm also hoping that some of the ways I found to take care of myself might work for you too.

I haven't seen too many stories or articles about women of color who have dealt with breast cancer issues.

Yes, this is truly a disease that doesn't care what the color of your skin is. However, did any of your doctors tell you what to do to minimize the chance of keloids? Did they even ask if you or anyone in your family was prone to this type of scar tissue? Or what kind of product you could use after the surgeries to try to get your skin close to the color it was before?

Some of what I have to say really applies to women of all races, but I felt that somehow, someone might want to hear what an average, middle aged, single parent women of color went through in the working world and the struggles of trying to raise a young child in the midst of an illness that most don't think about that much until it strikes close to home. And just maybe they can relate to some of it.

Not by any means are these words of an expert.

I am just a common everyday person that found affordable solutions for some of the things I was going through. And some of the ways I dealt with the mental anguish of my disease and illness in a world that was oftentimes cruel and dispassionate.

If no one ever reads this but my sisters, then I will still be blessed, because if they read it, I have fulfilled a promise I made to them and myself many years ago.

I'm going to tell you how this started, the battles, the triumph, and how I overcame this breast cancer. And hopefully not in a seriously boring way.

I'm going to write this the way I talk. I am not worried if it's not grammatically correct. Yes, I split infinitives, and used verbs wrong sometimes, but that's how I talk. I don't think about proper English when I'm talking to someone. I want it to be readable and understandable. So I'm not doing it like a library book or periodical. I'm doing it my way.

I did not lie or fabricate any of the things you're going to read. I know that at times that I actually down played some of the treatment that I received while going through this long illness. Because I'm not out to hurt anyone, I'm just telling it like it was and in some aspects still is for some of us. I know it is for me.

I sent a copy of my first few pages to my sisters, and one of them told me that I didn't say enough about what I went through. But, I'm not trying to talk as much about the way I was treated. I want to talk about how I survived.

If some people are offended, maybe it will be because they know deep down that no person deserved to be talked to or treated the way that I was. And I hope that they will understand just how detrimental it can be. Maybe just maybe, something I say will make a difference.

And I'll have no problem facing anyone who feels that I've done them wrong. What's that old saying? "If the shoe fits." If anyone is offended by what I've written, maybe they will actually think about why they feel that way.

For those of you with children, remember how you treated them when they didn't feel good. Even something like a stomach ache or a cold. You hurt for them and just wanted so much for them to be okay. Some of you even wishing that it were you instead of them that was sick.

When someone is sick, treat them that way. Not with pity, but with concern and maybe even a little compassion. It really does make a difference. Try to believe them. They may be sicker than you think.

And ladies, if you feel sick, don't give up just because that doctor doesn't believe you. Keep going until you find someone that does. Or, one that can show you proof that you're not sick.

I believe that at times our society has automatically deemed us, women, second-class citizens. And I've lived in countries where that is actually true. One country where women were considered even less than second class. Women of color are often, in my opinion, treated worse than that.

You do not have to allow anyone to treat you that way. Become the first class women that you are, you have a right to expect respectful treatment. You have the right to demand it. Not in a mean or nasty way, but through perseverance and faith. Don't let anyone bring or keep you down.

You have a tough enough battle ahead, dealing with your illness. Don't let people be the obstacle that keeps you from doing what you need to do to make it through this.

And don't you be an obstacle to yourself. You really can be your own worst enemy.

You have a right to be as healthy and happy as you can be. Both mind, body, and spirit.

And so the battle begins

March 2002, can I remember exactly what day, no. Why is it important to me, because one day that month, in that year, my entire life as I knew it changed, forever. And I didn't have any idea of what a life change it would be.

I hadn't been in Georgia very long. When my sister's husband was stationed here, in 1998, she asked me if I would let my son move here and go to school with my nephew. So in 1999, I agreed and he moved without me. I visited every three months, but I couldn't stand it, so in 2000, I quit my job in upstate New York, and moved down here to be with him again. It was also the first time that all three sisters had lived in the same state since we left home. It was the base that I started my military career at, so I was okay with moving back to a place I had lived before.

So, in March of 2002, a military friend of my sisters' family was retiring. My sister, nephew and I went together. It's a very formal affair at times, with a lot of standing. I can't even remember what we were standing for, the national anthem, presentation of an award, or the American flag. Something.

When I stood up, I immediately popped out in a sweat, became nauseous, dizzy and swayed. I remember that everything went white. I grabbed my nephew and he held me up until we could sit down again.

For the next almost year and a half I struggled. Back and forth to the doctor. Working every day, until I was physically drained. Back to the doctor on days I could barely move or think straight. Trying to self diagnose because blood tests, ENT appointments, nothing showed anything seriously wrong. So I was told.

Finally reaching the point where I was beginning to believe it was all psychological. Had to be. They were doctors; they had to know what was up. Since they weren't finding anything, it just had to be all in my mind.

Sometimes a little anemic, other times vitamin deficient, but no big deal, you'll be okay. That's what the doctor would sometimes say. Headaches so bad that I had to lie in bed with the covers over my head and not move so that I wouldn't throw up or pass out.

Migraines, NO, stress because you're a single parent, working every day, and not raising your child the way family and even some friends think you should. These were all things that were going through my mind, since the doctors insisted that I was not ill.

Then I started bleeding. I tried to wish it away because the same thing had happened before, years ago, and a doctor told me I could stop it any time I wanted to. It was all in my head. Really don't think that's where the blood was coming from, but........

The first time this happened, after two months of bleeding they found that I had an ectopic pregnancy. Put me in the hospital and the doctor said and I quote "if you don't die tonight, we'll operate in the morning." As soon as they cut me open, the tube exploded and I lost the baby and one of my fallopian tubes.

So imagine how I felt going through this again. The bleeding started April 16, 2003. I went to the doctor in May. After 22 days of bleeding, and 7 days of estrogen pills, the bleeding stopped.

At the time, I had a primary doctor that really thought I was faking a lot of my symptoms. Let me say that I insisted on seeing a different doctor then the one that had told me to stop always thinking that I was ill. And thankfully, I did see someone else because she wasn't there when I went in for the bleeding or for my follow up.

Three days after the bleeding stopped, it started again. Back to the doctor. Thankfully again my primary doctor wasn't there, so I got to see someone else. I didn't get to see the doctor that gave me the estrogen pills; I was assigned a different doctor. And he actually believed that something was wrong, because even after the bleeding stopped, the other symptoms did not.

A battery of blood tests, not like I wasn't losing enough already, I had to give more. Also, a mammogram and pap smear. I had managed to avoid these most of my career.

In June, I had the mammogram. "You have lumpy breasts and a calcified mass." Okay, no big deal. Many of us have lumpy breasts. So I wasn't in the least concerned about the lumps. I've had cysts since I started developing. I would just wait for them to burst open, and then I'd clean them out with peroxide or alcohol, and keep on going. Only when they got too big or I couldn't get everything out of them myself would I go to the doctor and have them cut. None of the cyst was ever biopsied or sent off to pathology for testing.

Mind you, getting those cysts cut was something I tried to avoid, because there was no way to numb the area. That's what I was told anyway. Imagine someone putting a cigarette out on your boob, and that's the intense sort of pain you feel when they cut that bad boy open. And they always said things like, "this will sting a little." Okay, right, I've had bee stings before but never did it feel like someone set my chest on fire.

I was actually in one place where the doctor got so tired of seeing me that he gave me a scalpel and told me to do it myself.

Did I mention that when I was finally allowed to see a civilian doctor, he would numb the area before he cut. It didn't stop the pain, but it was a lot less severe. Imagine that.

So, the mammogram was considered abnormal. Lumps and a small mass of unspecified cells. My new primary doctor decided I needed an ultrasound. The ultrasound showed micro calcifications, so he then decided on a biopsy.

The surgeon decided to do the ABBI procedure. Of course, I had no idea what this was.

I did the pre-op on the 25th of June. No big deal, they stuck my breast in this hole, marked it with the wonderful blue ink and home I go to wait. Got some pills to take the night before and the morning of the procedure, to help me relax.

Was I nervous, yes, scared, no, because it's just a simple procedure that I wouldn't be put to sleep for. And the surgeon said that this type of calcification had a 90% non cancerous rate. The lumps after all were just more cysts, so no need to worry.

The pills the night before did absolutely nothing for me. I had a hard time sleeping, but chalked it up to the fact that for the last year and a half I was lucky to sleep four hours a night. That had become my norm. What worried me was the fact that the pills didn't help me relax.

When I got up the next morning to get ready, I had two more pills to take. I was very anxious because the pills the night before didn't do anything. So I was thinking that these wouldn't work either.

Let me tell you, within fifteen minutes I was high as a kite.

Here's what I remember

Giggling about how drugged up I was. Not the least bit worried about what was about to happen. I was feeling good.

I do remember getting in to the car. Then all of the sudden we were at the hospital.

Hospital room? Don't remember too much about that ride. Veda helping me undress. I think my clothes actually took themselves off.

Walking with a nurse to the procedure room. I know that my feet did not touch the ground.

Lying on my stomach with my breast in this hole. There was only one hole, but I didn't feel the other breast being smashed.

Staring at a wall. Somebody was talking; don't ask me what they said. They could have asked me anything they wanted to and I would have told them. It was as if I had taken some sort of truth serum.

Seeing Veda waiting for me when the nurse walked me back to the waiting room. My clothes came back on by themselves too. Wow!

Walking to the car. Going to bed. Don't even ask, cause I have no idea how that happened.

Not a lot of pain, because I took those pills on schedule, whether I thought I needed them or not. I wasn't taking any chances. Plus, I was legally high and knew I wouldn't have a hangover the next day. Gotta love it!

Even though big sis, Veda, was moving to a foreign country, which involved so much work, she was there to take me to the hospital. My son was staying with her family in the hotel. They had already moved out of their home.

Follow up:

On the 7th of July, I had my follow up to make sure that I was healing okay. Now this is when I was sure that I had the right surgeon.

He walked through the door with tears in his eyes and said, "You have BREAST CANCER." I don't know who was more shocked.

Denial was the first thing I felt. "I did not just hear that. No way, not me."

"Death sentence" was my second thought. What's going to happen to my child?

Was it fear? I honestly don't know. I was confused, refusing to believe this could happen to me. Trying to figure out what to do with a stubborn, rebellious, yet loving, caring, normal 14 year old son who may have to grow up without his Mom. His Dad walked away from us when he was only three years old and now I felt as if I was deserting him too.

Mind you, all of this was going through my head even as I sat in the doctors' office while he tried to explain what DCIS, was and what he was going to do next.

Ductal what? Is that even English?

I looked at the pamphlet with him, listened to every word he said. Going to have to take the calcified area and a small amount of the healthy tissue area around it so that we're sure we got it all. Don't think we'll have to touch the lymph nodes because the cancer has not broken through the duct yet. That was supposed to be a good thing. Of course, I'm thinking, how can any kind of breast cancer be a good thing?

Walked out to the nurses' station, waited while they made the necessary appointments for CAT scans, bone scans and then surgery.

So much to do before all of this surgery actually happens. .

Back to the base to tell my doctor what was going on. He worked very hard through numerous obstacles to try to figure out what was wrong with me. He had fought hard to find out what was going on. He took me out of work that day. I remember asking him if it was alright to be sick now. He just looked at me and said "Yes". He called my sickness, cancer related fatigue. After all this time of feeling so bad, I didn't have a clue that cancer could have had anything to do with being so sick. Cancer related fatigue. Look it up. It's a trip. No one told me about it, so even though the doctor said it was okay to be sick, I wasn't convinced.

So if you end up with this disease, read up on cancer related fatigue. CRF. You may have been ill for a long time and not even have realized it. After a while, I did realize that it was okay to be sick. That what I was going through was legitimate. Did that diagnosis help? Yes and no.

Yes, because I finally knew that it was okay to feel the way I felt.

No, because I still felt that that was not all that was wrong.

Now that I knew that I was sick, the roller coaster of emotions was just as bad as the disease itself.

Still 7 July, and now I have to go to the hotel and tell my son and my family what has happened. Mind you that my sister and her family are only days away from leaving. Without them here the nearest family is a three hour drive away.

The shock and fear on their faces still did not bring me to tears. We held hands and prayed. Then we hugged and life went on. My brother in law left a few days later, sister and nephew still had to wait for paperwork and visas. Joshua, my son, stayed with them in the hotel so that I could go to appointments and get things together before the surgery.

I also think that because my son Joshua and my nephew Terry were so close, that he stayed with them so that he could talk and be a child a little while longer. The boys had spent a lot of time together over the years and acted more like brothers than cousins.

And I think that my sister was trying to give me time to deal with my own thoughts and feelings as much as possible, without worrying that my son would be okay.

I don't know if they ever talked about the cancer with him, I've never asked. But Joshua is just as stubborn as I am, so if they tried, I would be surprised if he told them anything. Very grateful if he did. It took years before he and I even talked about my cancer.

So if you have family, ask them if they want to talk. But if they don't, if there not ready, try to understand and let them come to you when they are ready. Trying to force someone to talk, may only cause them to shut down when you need them the most.

I think that also applies to everyone in your life. Some of my friends at first let me bring it up. They didn't try to get me to talk about it; they waited for me to say something.

Give everyone time to deal with it in their own way. You had to, and so do they!

Now, I'm sure we all know some noisy folk. And they tried to get me to give out details from day one. Some wanted to know some very personal things; I just had to tell them that I didn't want to talk about it. Not in a nasty way, but firm enough that they got the point.

You could tell that they just wanted something else to gossip about, and I was bound and determined that it wasn't going to be me.

Don't be afraid to tell them that you don't feel like talking about it. If they don't respect your feelings, you may need to reevaluate that relationship.

Now that you know how it started, let me tell you what this whole story is really about.

What I really want to talk about is how I dealt with the loneliness of this disease. Some of the ways I found to take care of my skin, my hair, my body. And most importantly how I learned to deal with and eventually, heal my mind and spirit.

Find good doctors

This to me is by far the most important thing you can do for yourself, in my opinion.

Being in the military at the time, I really thought that I had no choice of doctors. You were assigned a doctor according to what unit you were in, and that's who you saw. So, I battled with one who was absolutely obnoxious to me at times.

I went through three primary care doctors before I was diagnosed with breast cancer. I consider myself lucky that when I started bleeding my primary doctor was not there. That's when I saw a doctor that believed me and put me on the estrogen pills. Unfortunately, I didn't get to see her to many times before I was assigned another doctor. He is the one that ordered the blood tests, mammogram and told me that he believed something was wrong, and that he wouldn't give up until he found out what it was.

Hearsay has it that he got in a lot of trouble for all of the effort he put into helping me. And I believe it because the doctors only had a limited amount of time to spend with each patient. Treat the symptoms without really putting too much effort into finding the cause, seemed to me to be the way things were being done. When I went to see him, he took his time and that was unacceptable. He ordered tests that his superiors often felt were an unnecessary expense.

He guarded my privacy when people who had no business tried to get in to my medical records. He actually protected me as much as he could.

Eventually, he left, but thankfully not while I was going through my cancer treatments. He took care of me the way few doctors during my career ever had. And I'll forever be grateful to him for that.

Believe it or not, after he left, I was assigned the same doctor that told me to stop thinking that I was sick. I had, I thought, no choice. She treated me with disdain and disgust whenever I went in, so even when I was considered cancer free, I still had other issues, but I would go in only when I couldn't take it anymore. I suffered with her again until an incident came up with my toe. That's in here later on.

I absolutely refused to see her again after that.

My oncologist was outstanding. He listened; we talked and he answered any questions I had. I did not know much, but I felt that he tried to help me the best he could. Chemotherapy was considered, but he felt that I would be okay without it. We considered all of the facts and decided not to do it. Since I had estrogen receptive breast cancer, hormone therapy was out of the question. He gave me diet suggestions, even told me about natural foods and different ways to deal with the effects of the radiation and then the tamoxifan drug that I would be taking when radiation treatments were finished. And he was a Christian, so we often talked about prayer and how that could affect my treatment and recovery. He was such a comfort to me; I actually enjoyed going to see him. And man would he go off on me if he felt that I wasn't doing something right. He or one of his nurses would call if he didn't like the way I looked after an appointment. Or just to check up on me between appointments.

My radiologist was okay. He wasn't much of a people person in my opinion, but he was good at what he did, I felt. He had that air of super intelligence that I liked. And he wasn't overbearing or mean. I saw more of his nurses then I did him, so I was okay with it. They were wonderful.

Now my first plastic surgeon visit. What can I say? Nightmare comes to mind. Can't tell you how I really felt and keep this g-rated., when I think about that day. I have a tendency to develop keloids. It's mainly a woman of color thing, where our scar tissue builds up on the skin as we heal. The first plastic surgeon I was sent to examined me and told me how he would do the surgery. When I asked him about the keloids, he shrugged me off and said that he didn't worry about that. It was no big deal to him.

I went right back to my primary doctor and told him that I refused to have that man touch me. My oncologist wanted me to see a specialist in Atlanta because of the cystic issue and the keloids anyway. So after another year long battle I was finally allowed to go. He was a specialist in his field and did the best he could with what he was allowed to do. After my breast reduction, during one of my follow up examinations, he found a suspicious lump that he wanted to biopsy right away. I went outside made the necessary phone calls to my clinic, over 90 miles down the road, went back in, got admitted and biopsied, then left and went to the airport to go on a business trip. Now mind you I did what I was supposed to do, however, weeks later it was deemed an unnecessary procedure by the powers that be and I ended up having to foot the bill.

Okay, getting to the point. If you don't like you're doctor, find a new one. You have got to feel comfortable with the people that you are going to be seeing for months and years to come. I had several opinions before I consented to the surgeries and radiation.

Read and study as much as you can. If you can't ask your doctor a question and get an answer, that's a problem. You might not have the right doctor. Do not give up if you have concerns about any aspect of your treatment. It's your body and you have every right to know anything and everything that's going on and what you can expect to happen. As much as possible. Sometimes you may feel like you don't really want to know, I felt that way, but in the end I'm glad I did read some and ask questions.

Research the doctors you're going to. Ask you primary doctor what he knows about the others doctors that you're going to be sent to. Look them up on the internet. There are several tools out there, use them. Find out as much as you can before your appointment. If you don't have a computer, libraries do. Take the time it's worth it.

Write down questions you want to ask. I kept, and still do, notepads all over my house, because I'll think of something and not remember it later on. I keep them in my purse too.

I would go to the doctor, then come home and call my sister. She always asked a question that I had no answer to. Always.

The only stupid question is the one you don't ask. I learned that the hard way also.

Insist, I can't stress this enough, insist, on getting a copy of your medical records. Or at least take the time to read them. They may be private, but you have a right to see them. Don't let anyone tell you that you don't. They need to be accessible to you any time you want.

When I first joined the military, they used to purge the medical records and throw away what they felt was unnecessary. Doing that, I think I lost a lot of important information that could have helped me now. One volume of my records actually disappeared, or so I was told when I tried to get copies. So when I re-joined, I started asking for copies every six months. You'd be surprised what's not there.

If I saw a civilian doctor, I would ask for my own copies of what they were doing. Many times that information was not in my base records. Sometimes, the civilian doctors' just didn't send it.

My surgeon, radiologist and oncologist didn't know each other, so it helped to be able to let them know what each of them was doing. And of course my primary doctor did not have any way to know what was going on without getting copies from the off base doctors.

So whatever you do, whether you are military or not, be sure that you have copies that you can keep safe at home. It will also help when you start going to different doctors. They don't always know each other and you may need to show them what you had done before.

Just cut it OFF.

My hair had started breaking and falling out during the year and a half prior to the breast cancer diagnosis.

My hair dresser called it stress, and I believe that some of it was that. But my body chemistry was all screwed up, and I think that was part of it too. And after the surgeries and radiation treatments, it just started looking really ratty no matter what I did.

It was dry, brittle, lots of split ends and short patchy spots.

I was still taking care of my hair the way I always had. I didn't have the extra money to go to the hairdresser every week, so I did it at home. Never had big problems before, I self permed, conditioned, and didn't use a lot of heat. I enjoyed pulling it back and throwing on a hair piece. It was convenient and I liked being able to change my look.

Keeping my hair during my illness and treatments was a huge battle. It was so important to me not to cut my hair. I did cry sometimes when I combed it and clumps came out in my hands. But I kept it long because I refused to believe that I couldn't take care of it myself. I was not going to give up my "mane" without a fight. Ponytails and hair pieces were like a trademark of mine.

Okay, if you're not a woman of color, how politically correct is that, you may not understand this part. I washed my hair once a week. It was a ritual for me to wash, condition, grease the scalp, the whole deal. But once I got sick, it was sometimes just too hard for me to do. May not sound like such a big deal, but I sometimes could not stand up in the shower that long without getting weak and dizzy. And if I tried to do it in the sink, I might have a dizzy spell or even what I call a "white out." So it became increasingly hard to do. And like I said before, I couldn't afford to go to the hairdresser every week.

I tried getting it braided, but that just helped it break off even more. And I couldn't stand to leave the braids in longer than two weeks. I didn't like to tie my hair at night, sisters head needed to breathe. And if I covered my head I got to hot. So braids just didn't last very long.

A few months after my radiation treatments ended I just couldn't take it anymore. It wasn't falling out anymore, but it was just so broken off and dry. So, I went to the hair dresser and said, cut it off. I cried again, but I couldn't stand losing it like that. I wore it natural until it grew to the point that it was out of control. By then, I felt like I could take good care of it again.

What I'm trying to say is, if I had to do it all again, I would have cut it sooner and kept it short throughout the whole ordeal. Not only was it easier to take care of. Wash, condition, oil the scalp and air dry, it took away some of the stress level.

Believe it or not, something that simple did relieve some of the stress of everyday. Didn't matter if I didn't feel like doing my hair, I could just comb it and go.

And it grew back. I've even cut it a few times since then. But if it had not grown back, I would have been okay. I realized that my beauty, or what I thought of at the time as beauty, was not what I looked like on the outside.

I stopped worrying about how my hair looked and concentrated on living day to day.

Sounds a little shallow, but I think that sometimes we become obsessed with the outer look and don't spend enough time with what really matters. Your inner health and well being. To me that's where your true beauty shines.

I've seen some beautiful women of all colors with little or no hair. Your true inner beauty can shine through because of who you are and how you present yourself. With, or without hair. And if you don't feel that way, they make some really beautiful, comfortable wigs, hats and scarves.

Does anyone else smell that?

Remember when the doctor said; don't get your breast wet? I just kind of looked at him like, what are you talking about? How am I supposed to clean my body if I have to take a shower with my back to the water? I was thinking my breasts aren't' the only thing up front that needs washing you know. And I liked to wash my hair in the shower.

Well, I learned how to take that shower without getting to wet. Standing with my back to the water and not soaping that area at all. I figured that the nurses and doctors were used to the funk. No one actually ever said that I stank, and maybe the radiation killed the smell, who knows. Not the first one to do this, and not the last.

And no deodorant under that arm? You're kidding right? Well, it wasn't a joke, but it was very hard to go out in public without that. Amazing the things you take for granted until you can't do them anymore.

Having had to sometimes live in a house with no indoor plumbing growing up, we had water in the kitchen sink, but that was it, I learned how to do what we call "cat baths." Making sure that the necessary areas were washed. I'd be more specific, but I think you know what "necessary areas" means. Sometimes you may not have the energy to stand in that shower, it's okay. Do the cat bath thing and keep on rolling. Or if you can afford it, buy a bath seat. I found that difficult, because I couldn't keep the water off my chest as well as if I just stood up.

Some things were elemental. When I permed my hair, I always washed it out at the kitchen sink. So that just meant using the sink for normal hair washing also. Sometimes I could even afford to go to my hairdresser. If you can't afford to, try to find a friend who will be willing to come over and wash it for you once in a while. That didn't happen for me. Or, like I said before, make it easy on yourself, cut it. Short hair is easier to care for if you wear it natural or just get a texturizor or something like that.

When treatment is over, you have to still be careful with what you put on the affected area. The best thing I did was go out and get some pure soap. Well, as pure as possible. I love body wash, but I think I healed better not putting perfumed soap on my breast area. I did this for about a year after the partial mastectomy, the reduction, and each time I had a cyst removed. Now, I used my body wash everywhere else, love that smell and feel, but not on my breast until I was good and sure that it healed and didn't hurt too much to touch.

And instead of a wash cloth, I used a bath sponge. It wasn't as abrasive on the skin. If I was overly sensitive at times, I just used my hand. I'm not embarrassed to say that. While I was having the different surgeries and even after radiation, sometimes it was too painful to wash the "normal" way. No cloth or sponge in the world was soft enough not to hurt.

The radiation was like a laser treatment to me. Never been a hairy person, but now I didn't have to shave under that arm like I used to. Think of it this way, it helps the razor last longer.

Hmm, something positive to come out of this experience after all.

Get to a dentist

No one told me until I was cancer free that proper dental care was important. I went for an annual exam and when the hygienist found out that I had had cancer, she asked me if I had used any special toothpaste or rinse. I was floored. I had no idea that my teeth and gums could be affected by radiation to my breast.

I was thinking at the time, here we go again, something else no one told me.

I did have gum issues before the cancer, but I took care of my teeth the best I could. Never had a cavity until I was in a car accident years before. My mouth was wired for eight weeks and all I could do was brush the fronts of my teeth and rinse. I ended up with three surface cavities and was devastated because I was the first female in my family to have cavities.

This may seem shallow too, but like I said before, we grew up sometimes without indoor plumbing, but we always brushed our teeth. Mom was not having funky breath.

The hygienist was so sweet, she worked with me every three months to get my teeth and gums back into shape. It was thankfully not too late.

So, find a dentist and make sure that you keep going. I have a civilian dentist now, and she and her wonderful office staff have taken over keeping my teeth and gums healthy. Find one that will work with you, and keep that smile!

And I'll say that just like with the doctors, if you are not comfortable with one, shop around until you find a dentist that you can be comfortable with. I'm not opening my mouth to someone I can't be comfortable around.

Even if you have dentures or partials, it's important to go to the dentist. You don't know what's going to happen to your gums or bones. Please take the time to find out.

What has happened
to my skin?

Man, did I struggle with this. Many days I would be out and look down at my arms or hands and think, "I look like Caspar." When did that happen?

First of all, we all know that lotion is a must. I don't care what color you are, you need to not be ashy. I don't know about you, but I have very innocently offered lotion to people I've seen that needed it.

During my illness and subsequent radiation treatments, my skin was off the chain.

Now, I could not afford those fancy crèmes and lotions, so what did I do? Dollar stores baby. Petroleum jelly, cocoa butter lotions, baby oil, and baby oil gels. They worked just as good as spending $50 on a tube or jar of something with a fancy name or smell. I am not nor have I ever been a slave to labels. If it works, I don't care where it comes from or who made it.

If you take the time to look at the ingredients, you'll see that most lotions and crèmes start off with water anyway, so why spend that kind of money if you don't have to. I personally just didn't think it was necessary for me. As long as it worked, that's all I was concerned with.

Since my body soaked up baby oil like I soak up water, I'm a water freak; I didn't use it that much. Baby oil gel lasted longer, but for me, good old fashioned petroleum jelly worked the best. Every day!

I've never worn a lot of makeup. If I did, I took it off with petroleum jelly and cotton balls. To wash my face I used a white wash cloth and hot water. Even now, I seldom use soap or any kind of facial wash. I have very sensitive skin, but I did find one brand of face wash that wouldn't break me out as much. I used it about once a week. And a very thin layer of petroleum jelly was my night time moisturizer. Most of the time I just washed my face and let it breathe.

I also scrubbed my lips at night and put on a layer of Vaseline or carmex or this vitamin e crème in a tube that I found.

I found that after a few weeks of radiation, my skin seemed to as stay dry as the Mojave Desert, so I greased up several times a day, and stayed away from open flames. My feet and hands seemed to be the worst. So I bought some white ankle socks, also from my favorite dollar store, and I greased my feet every night before I went to bed and wore socks. A habit I continue to this day, because it works.

I loved getting manicures when I could. But during this time I just couldn't do it, so I found ways to do it myself. I had learned how to do manicures from a friend of mine while stationed in California. So that was no big deal. I always try to keep my hands in good shape.

Now the feet, that's another story. I had never gotten pedicures very often to begin with. Don't really care for people messing with them that much.

My mother used to soak her feet at home. She had very bad feet and she did it to relieve the pain. I learned from that. And let me tell you that dish detergent works wonderfully. I would fill a pail with the hottest water I could stand and squirt in that dish detergent then just sit back and relax until the water got cold. Sometimes I would use Epsom salt or bubble bath.

It sounds so simple, and it is. But it feels so good. Try it you might like it.

My radiologist told me not to put anything on the breast while I was being radiated. Anything you use may have chemicals that could cause problems with the process.

And with my tendency to develop cysts, we didn't want to risk adding that complication. So I didn't do anything until treatments were over. I suffered second and third degree burns, even while using the cream that the doctor supplies. By the way, ask about the cream at your first appointment with the radiologist. You might not need it for the first week or so, but ask anyway. I didn't even know about it. One of my other doctors asked me if I had received it, that's how I found out.

Even though it was painful, I started using cocoa butter cream with vitamin e in it about a week after the radiation treatments ended. My breast looked like a piece of burnt toast and felt like a baked piece of meatloaf. Lumpy and burnt. Sister wasn't having that.

It took a while but the cream did eventually help my skin return to a color close to the rest of my body.

And if you're like me, you need to learn not to worry too much about the skin peeling off. Did it hurt, DAH? But that was part of the healing process. Remember, you've just been radiated, that's poison. So think of the peeling like a piece of fruit or vegetable. Sometimes, you got to peel off the skin to get to the good part.

What do they say, no pain, no gain. Try to remember that when you go to bed and mistakenly turn over on your stomach. Not a good thing.

Forget the bra and please don't touch me

Sensitive is going to happen. Well it did to me anyway. I called it sensitive but really for me it was more pain. If anyone brushed me by mistake, or when I was trying to wash up, it hurt.

I stopped wearing a bra before the partial mastectomy. I did wear a sports bra when I was going out in public, but at home, I released the puppies and let them breath. And I bought some what we call "wife beater" t-shirts to wear under my shirts. Okay for those of you who might not know what that is, it's athletic t-shirts.

I found the cotton very cool and not abrasive. Even though they touched my skin, it didn't hurt as much as wearing a bra did. I'm sure silk would have felt the same way, but I do most of my shopping at the "Marts" and stores that have "Dollar" in them, not so much at the high end stores.

I slept in those t-shirts many nights.

One of my friends gave me a very large silky feeling t-shirt. It was sort of a mesh fabric, and it felt so good. I also wore that some nights and some days until my son came home.

The more air I could get on my chest, the better it felt.

I bought shirts at least a size bigger than I was at the time. And if they don't tell you, you need to get some button down shirts more than pullovers. It was just so much easier to not have to lift my arm over my head. And after a while it actually didn't feel that great lifting my arm that high. Plus, you're going to be undressing more than a stripper on a Saturday night.

So to me it was about being as comfortable as possible, in an uncomfortable situation.

And let me tell you, good bras are very important. When you start wearing one again, spend some money on them. I can actually feel the difference between a cheap bra and an expensive one.

There are some stores that will measure you. If you can't do that, I couldn't, find someone you trust to measure you so that you'll be sure to get the right size.

I do very little under wire now, because it still tends to fit me the wrong way and hurt. So I do go out and pay some money for better bras. Worth the price!

The doctor told me to massage my breast after my surgery. I ended up with a buildup of scar tissue on the inside, and we were hoping that this would help reduce it. And that scar tissue just happened to be where the under wire hit.

It did help a little, but I still had to have a very large piece of it surgically removed. Hopefully that won't happen to you.

Do the massage thing. I did not enjoy doing that to myself, however, it did break up some of the scar tissue and my breast was not as hard as it was after the radiation treatments and surgeries were over.

Who knows, maybe some of you will be lucky enough to find someone to do it for you!

Thicken your skin.

Of course I don't mean literally.

Although after months of MRI's, x-rays, ultrasounds, operations, and then radiation, I was wishing my boob was made of leather. Maybe that way I wouldn't have been able to feel the pain. For those of you who lost your breast, I'm sorry, but believe it or not , sometimes I wondered if that might have been an easier thing to do. I didn't have that option, but I thought about it a lot.

I mean thicken your mental skin.

Strangers will mark your body. I had blue ink from my neck to my navel. Sometimes I wondered just where that treasure map was going to lead. It was just so comfortable wearing turtle necks and collared shirts in the Georgia heat and humidity. Yea right. But if I didn't, eventually, someone was going to ask me what those blue marks were on my neck. So, I chose to cover rather than be questioned all of the time.

They will poke your boobs, stick needles in your boobs, mark you with marker and pens, and remember all of those wonderful hands on exams. Sometimes I felt like that one person had at least four hands. There were just too many fingers. I got felt so many times that I know if I hadn't been sick I would have loved it. Woo hoo, all those hands. How many of us can say they've been felt up by that many men. Legally? Now, I ain't ever gonna say that I enjoyed having women touching me. Can't swing from that tree baby, but if it's your thing, so be it. I've never been an exhibitionist, but I got to the point where taking off my shirt in front of strangers was no big deal. "You want to bring in a medical student, okay, come on in and bring a friend."

And I know that all of those machines were made by men. No women in her right mind would invent a machine that takes your boob and squishes it to the size of a dollar pancake. Or uses so much gel that by the time they finish the ultrasound you feel like you've put the KY jelly in the wrong place.

At first it felt like I was part of a carnival side show, but after a while I realized that these doctors and nurses see so much of this that it's no big deal to them. That's when it became no big deal to me. Even when one of my boobs looked like a softball, felt like a hardball, and the other a watermelon, I still just didn't care when it came time for exams. I'd flash you like I was getting paid to do it.

Of course I realize now that I should have been paying them for having to see that mess.

And people, wonderful, beautiful, unbelievable. PEOPLE.

They are going to say things that will blow you away. I could not believe some of the things that came out of their mouths. My feelings were hurt too many times to count. I felt like a whipping board. Try not to think of it as anything. They will not understand that not only is your body fragile, but also, your mind. And things that may not have hurt you in the past will become huge. When you look back on it, you might feel like I do now, they just didn't know what to say or how to deal with what was happening. And that the situation I was going through just made me overly sensitive to some things.

I know it was hard on my sisters, and my female friends. I wasn't thinking about that at the time though.

Some of my female friends looked at me like they were afraid it was catching. And many times they were just at a loss for words. It was like, since I had cancer they didn't know what to say to me. Normal conversations that we used to have about any and everything just didn't happen.

And men, oh boy. Some of the guys I knew were afraid to touch me or even look me in the eyes. I could see them looking sometimes trying to figure out which breast it was. Or saying hello, then looking down at the floor like they dropped something.

The man I cared about, at that time, hurt me several times.

First, when I told him about the cancer. I felt that there was no one to take care of Joshua should I die, and he said "I don't know what the problems are with you and your sister, but you know she'll take care of your son."

POW! Not the words of someone that you really wanted to be understanding and compassionate.

Okay, so you're expecting me to die. That's what I was saying to myself. I was expecting, maybe I should say, wishing that he would have said, "Baby everything will be alright, you'll be fine."

I had only been in Georgia two years prior to the cancer, but the lack of concern from the office I worked in still shocked me. I was only visited by three people in my office. My supervisor, my commander, and a co-worker. The day I left work, I was all but forgotten. As a matter of fact, they actually tried to find a way to get rid of me, so I've been told. And I believe it. I'm glad I didn't know that until much later. It would have been so much more hurtful and I believe detrimental to my already weak body and mind.

But lying on the sofa, day after day, totally alone, was for me one of the hardest parts of being sick. I felt like I was on another planet. Exiled by my people to die. Okay, okay, a little overly dramatic. But seriously, that was one of the loneliest times of my life.

The only two people in my organization that showed any kind of interest in my son and I's lives, I didn't even directly work for. Every few weeks I had to take a leave form in to get signed. Had to have permission to be on sick leave.

The first time I went to get my form signed, one very special man asked me how my son was doing. He said, bring him with you sometime. The next time I went in, I did. He took Joshua into another room and talked to him. The first time that happened I was shocked, but then after that I tried to make every effort to bring Josh with me so that he could have that male bonding time. Someone was actually taking the time out of there extremely busy schedule to talk to and listen to my son. And he so needed that, since there was no man at home or family close by.

The other was a very high ranking female in my organization. Whenever and wherever she saw me, she hugged me and asked me if I was alright. We talked several times during my ordeal, and she never made me feel like I wasn't important.

I will always be grateful for their kindness and compassion. To me they were what true leaders are all about.

So, if you don't get the compassion from your friends, family, co-workers, try to think of it this way. They just don't get it. And they can't because they are not you. Even those that have been through it can't understand what you may be feeling or not feeling, because we all have to deal with it in our own way.

And when you least expect it, what you or your family need may just come from the most unlikely people.

Those you expect it to come from or wanted it to come from may not understand that your emotions are as fragile as your body.

And you may also have to face the fact that some of them, just will not care.

Shoot, I didn't even get that for a while.

Now I won't lie, it took me years to realize some of these things. So while I was going through this disease, I was in a lot of turmoil. Constantly trying to figure out why people weren't calling or coming by. I was and still am a private person, but I could not understand how they could just not be bothered to check up on me or my son. I was a single parent going through a life threatening ordeal with no family close by. And in an organization that spoke of caring for your people, being a united front and showing concern for your well being and your family, it boggled the mind and changed the way I felt about my job and the people I worked with and for, for the rest of the time I was there.

Learn to smile. Sometimes it really will help you to feel better. It's going to be hard to do, but think of it this way. Those that care about you will really be happy to see you smiling. It will help them to think that you are doing and going to be okay.

I started smiling at people that got on my nerves. You know the old saying "kill them with kindness?" well, it really did work. Some people became very uneasy around me because I stopped letting them see that they were getting to me. I got some stupid comments from people because I was smiling, but they didn't care about what I was going through. So, I didn't want them to see or know just how I felt. What they sometimes thought was a smile, was really a smirk. Whatever works for you.

So, if you have to go it mostly alone, remember to depend on yourself. You truly are stronger than you think. And when the surgeries and treatments are over, you can say that you survived. And that's what really matters.

I can't go where or do what?

I was so sick. I sometimes think that the cancer was actually a blessing in disguise. Can't believe I just said that, but that's how I felt. It forced the doctors and the people I worked with to finally admit that something was actually wrong with me. They had to acknowledge that I was actually ill. HAH, some folks did not like having to admit that they were wrong about me. Some still don't.

During the year and a half that I struggled to find out what was going on, I found that I couldn't do some things anymore.

The one thing I could do was my job. I had been doing the same work for so many years, that it was a no brainer. And I think because I really enjoyed it so much and took pride in what I did; it was still easy to do.

Concentrating was the first thing that I started having trouble with. If someone was talking to me, at times I would just drift off. I would hear every other word or just not be able to listen at all.

I absolutely love to read. After a while, I would have to re-read the same sentence over and over, and still not get it. So I stopped. I kept buying books, hoping that one day I would be able get back that feeling. And I have.

I also loved to write. Poetry, songs. I was in my own world when I had a pen and paper. Even when I got a computer, I still liked to do it the old fashioned way.

Cooking is a passion of mine. We grew up all over the world, and even had a chance to live in or travel to several different foreign countries. I loved to watch people cook and then go home and try to figure out how to make that taste. I might not cook a lot all week long because of work, but we had to have that big Sunday dinner.

And don't get me started on music. I love any and all kinds of music. I spent so many hours just listening to music. Loved to sing, or try my hand at writing songs, making tapes and cd's. I even tried my hand at being a disc jockey.

I never liked to exercise that much, but I did try to keep in shape as much as I could. I forced myself to do it because I was in the military. I really wanted to be in better shape, and since I wasn't really sick, in their minds, I had to exercise.

All of this stopped or significantly slowed down, when I got sick.

I couldn't stand for very long without feeling like I was going to pass out. I was actually in physical pain, which later turned out to also be a legitimate issue. So, if I had to stand for a long time, the pain would cause me to become dizzy, pop out in a sweat and eventually pass out.

I had dizzy spells for no reason. And it didn't matter if I was driving, working. I could just be sitting around trying to relax and the room would start spinning, white spots would come in front of my eyes.

I prayed for sleep, but many nights, that just didn't come. So I was exhausted all of the time.

Eating was out of the question. I felt like I had morning sickness twenty four hours a day. I was nauseous all of the time. So that took care of me cooking a lot. Couldn't stand the smell of things I used to love to eat or cook.

Just understand that whatever you're going through you are very different now. If you can't do the things you enjoyed, or even the everyday things that you used to. It's okay.

My house didn't fall apart because I didn't clean it the way I used to. It wasn't as clean as I would have liked, it still isn't. But I did what I could when I could.

I stopped going out on Friday nights. I figured if I couldn't spend quality time at home with my son, I had no right to go out. Plus, after working all day, I very seldom felt like trying to go anywhere but home.

In time you just might feel like doing those things that you like to do again. And if you don't you may find that you've developed new hobbies or gifts.

Some things for me, took years to feel like doing again. And some things that I used to do, I had and still have no desire to do anymore.

So, try not to feel too guilty about the things you can't do while you're sick. You'll see this again, but it's worth saying many times. You are different, and you have a right to be.

Loneliness in my opinion is also a disease.

In my opinion and for me it is a disease I believe of the mind and spirit.

And no matter who you have around you, you may eventually feel a deep self pitying, soul wrenching, and gut twisting loneliness.

It is okay. I think it's normal. After all, have you ever been told that you have cancer before? Have you ever had to deal with your own mortality in that way?

My cancer was stage one ductal carcinoma in situ. Yes, I said stage one, which is a very low grade of cancer.

Now let me tell you how I feel about this stage thing. It's important yes, the earlier it's diagnosed, the better your chances of being saved are, but it's still all cancer. You have abnormal cells manifesting in your body. Something that if left untreated can be fatal. And even treatment and surgery does not always mean you are cured. So no matter what stage it is, you have the right to feel any way you want to.

However, back then, I felt that I had no right to feel bad because the doctors all said it wasn't a big deal. That it was low grade of cancer. Does what I've just said go with loneliness? To me it does, because it was a lonely feeling being sick and not being able to really talk about how I felt. I felt that if I did, I would be whining. Because I just wasn't supposed to be that sick.

If someone asked me how I felt, and I was honest, many times they would tell me to stop whining or complaining. So I tried not to let anyone know how scared and anxious I was all of the time. Or that I truly didn't feel well.

Then, there's the night. The time that you have to face yourself. My mind would not shut down. If sleep was not drug induced, and I don't take sleeping pills, now or then. So I spent many nights laying awake for hours thinking about what was happening to me.

The big "what if" was always on my mind.

What if surgery and radiation doesn't stop this?

What if they don't get it all?

What if I have to go back and have that breast removed and start all over?

What if it spreads before they do the surgery?

What if I die?

Then came the, "what wills."

What will I do if I lose my breast?

What will I do if they don't get it all the first time? Can I go through this and more again?

What will happen to my child if I die?

If you have ever felt like this, know that you are now alone. And I don't think that any doctor, family member, or friend, can give you the answers that you need. They can tell you what they think you should feel or how they think you should deal with your thoughts and feelings. But they are not you! In the end, only you can deal with what's happening and find a way to get through it.

But "Oh my goodness," can that loneliness sometimes feel like the darkest cloud hanging over you, or a weight laying on your chest that you can't get off.

Some call it loneliness, some depression, but whatever you choose to call it, find a way to deal with it or it can become so overwhelming that it will hinder your recovery. I considered it depression when I was having those pity parties. Not when I was just thinking about life and what could happen if things didn't work out okay.

Depression for me was more of a physical type of pain. Depression, I think broke my body down more. It sapped my strength, what little I had. But loneliness was more like an ache in my soul. It broke my spirit. You know how they say some people die from a broken heart. I believe it, and I also believe that the loneliness can do the same thing.

Whether you're married, in a relationship, or alone, find a sanctuary where you can go and think and deal with what's happening to you in your own way.

At the time I was going through this, I thought that having someone in my life would have helped me. Now I realize that, no, it would not have. I had a special friend, but we were just good friends. So even if he had been there for me, those nights alone would have happened anyway, after he fell asleep, or went out with the fellas, or just watched TV in the other room.

Though I was lonely, very often, I wanted to be alone. I did not want to go to my favorite hangout, not because I couldn't party or drink like I used to, but because I didn't feel like being stared at and I didn't want people feeling uncomfortable around me. I didn't want to go out to eat or go shopping and have people staring at the blue ink on my neck, or the breasts that were no longer the same size. Big shirts didn't hide everything.

How many times have people talked to your chest? Prior to my surgeries they did it because of how big I was; now, I felt that they did it trying to figure out which breast was smaller.

And I avoided direct eye contact. Even now, I can remember exactly why. I always felt ill. I was embarrassed for people to see me that way. While I was going through the surgeries and treatments, I felt like less of a woman, many days. I felt unworthy and not anything close to pretty, forget beautiful. I felt that my life was never going to be the same. Does any of this sound familiar?

Do I believe in God? Absolutely, I do believe in God. But for some reason, prayer did not comfort me, and after a while I stopped praying. I did not lose my faith. I just could not pray. I felt that since he knew my every thoughts and fears, that he could just read my mind and get it that way. I didn't feel like saying that prayer or asking him for help. He knew that's what I wanted. Why couldn't he just take care of it and make it go away.

Stop now, don't laugh. Even now sometimes I think "You know my thoughts, my hopes, and my dreams. Why can't you just read my mind?" But at least now I know it just doesn't work that way.

I hope that you will try to find something to believe in. God, Jehovah, Buddha, Muhammad, whatever or whoever. Find your spiritual self and hold on to it.

Even atheists believe.

If they didn't they wouldn't be atheist.

Do you or did you feel Guilty

I did.

Guilt consumed me. I felt that I had brought this on myself. I don't know how or why, but I spent a lot of time trying to figure out how this could happen to me.

I refused to believe that there was no way I could have prevented this. How did I cause this to happen to me?

I felt guilty because I didn't feel good. It had to be something that I was doing wrong. It had to be because of something that I had done. It had to be something that I could have controlled and changed.

Did my lifestyle cause this? What if I had tried to live a better life? Hadn't partied or stayed out late so much.

After constantly being told that there was nothing wrong with me, I felt guilty when I was too sick to go to work or to do the things that I did before. There had to be a way that I could wish away this disease. After all, to many times I had been told that it was all in my head.

Wrong body part!

When I found out I had breast cancer, I felt guilty because I didn't want to deal with it. I wanted to just lie down and not even try to fight. When my sisters and I started reading up on it, I just didn't want to do it. I wanted it to go away on its own. It was going to be too hard for me.

After all, it was only someone playing a cruel joke on me. Any day now, I was going to be told that it was a mistake. I'd be mad for a while, but I would get over it.

Guilty because it wasn't a stage four, it was only a stage one, so I shouldn't feel this bad. Too many other people were fighting for their lives with this disease. Some were not going to make it. Some would go through so much more than me.

I felt that I had no right to feel sorry for myself, but I couldn't help it.

Some of you may call it self pity. Some call it depression. I felt all of those things at times, but I truly believe that those feelings I just talked about were pure guilt.

It wasn't so much why me, or what if, or even why. It was more, what did I do to cause this and why couldn't I figure out what it was on my own.

Can you relate to this? I hope so, because I would hate to think that I really had lost my mind and just didn't know it.

We have so much to deal with, that people just can't help with. If I were rich, maybe I would have gone to a psychiatrist or therapist. But realistically, how many of us have those options?

I actually did see a psychiatrist on base, and he didn't feel that I was that bad. It was all chalked up to depression and I went off to a class to learn how to deal with it. Whoopee!

If you can afford the professional help, good for you. But if you can't, just let me say it again. It's okay to feel how you feel.

One day it will get better. Doesn't seem like it while you're going through it, but one day you'll wake up and you'll be okay.

It's okay to smile

You are going through one of the toughest battles you'll ever face. I wish you blessings and peace, as much as you can find.

These are some of the things that happened that helped me make it through:

My primary doctor was always telling me that I was going to be okay. That I would win this battle. He was very shocked when I told him about the cancer, but he was always available for me to talk to. And he even called a couple of times just to check on me. He believed that I was ill, and that I may not have always been treated responsibly, and he fought hard to find out what was wrong with me. He never gave up on me.

When the mammogram technician spotted the calcifications she was very compassionate. The doctor that read the films asked her to do it again. She came back in to the room, showed me the spots and said that she was sure that I would be okay. She was as gentle as possible with me and stopped if I told her that it hurt too much. After the partial and surgeries I saw her again. If I couldn't stand the pain, she would stop and let me rest and re-group.

Prior to my first procedure, I had to have an ultrasound. The female technician did the normal chitchat while she was doing her thing. When it was over, she actually hugged me and said I'm sorry. This stranger that I'd never met before or again. And days later, I received a get well card.

When I had the ABBI procedure and the surgeon came in with news of cancer, compassion was the first thing I saw on his face. I knew then that no one else would do my partial mastectomy. He had been the one to remove the cysts whenever I had to have them cut, and he was always aware of the pain I was going through.

The radiology nurses were so nice to me. One day when I came in and one of the nurses told me that she looked forward to me coming, even though it wasn't for a good reason. She said, you are always smiling, and we don't see too much of that in here. You make us feel good.

While I was getting prepped for treatment, she said that she and the other nurses also looked forward to seeing what kind of shoes I would have on that day.

My shoes had to match my shirt, pants or purse, always. I'm a shoe nut.

The plastic surgeon that did my breast reduction had my sister and I rolling, when he held up his hand and said, "This is how big you need to be, just enough to fit into my hand." We were not expecting that. Thankfully, he had big hands.

This is my favorite thing that happened. I laugh about it even now.

A very good female friend said something that I will never forget. I was so tired of fighting to have my breast reconstructed that I finally gave up. I was talking to her about the fact that I would never look the same because one breast was so misshapen. How could anyone want me this way? She said, "When is the last time a man asked you for some breast?" I did change the last word; breast is not the word she used. I laughed so hard, but you know what, she was right.

My point is that it may not seem like it while you're going through it, but something or someone is going to make you smile. Even during this most awful time of your life, you will laugh. They may not even realize that what they've said or done has made you feel better. Let them know. It just might matter to them.

And try to find a way to smile yourself. If you allow this disease to sap your being, it will. Try to remember that the battle is not just to get your body healthy.

Smile at the doctors and nurses. Smile at your spouse or children if you are blessed enough to have them. Smile at your neighbor, your friends, even a stranger. For a moment it will make you feel better.

Smile because you are still alive

Find something that comforts you

For me, I adopted a pet. She became my constant companion.

On days that I felt like I wasn't going to be able to do this much longer, I would come home and she would crawl up next to me on the sofa, and just lay there.

It was strange. She was a kitten, but instead of running around trying to play or get into everything, she came and stayed beside me.

Now, I'm no fool, I know that she was probably doing all of that ripping and running while I was out. That's why I closed off parts of the house, and limited her area.

But she seemed to sense that all I wanted was to rest when I got home from radiation treatments. Maybe she did it because she was tired by then too.

When my son came home, she would become a kitten again. They played and he took very good care of her. Feeding, cleaning the pan, making sure she had water.

Sometimes, Joshua and I would even play with her together.

So Spacey, named for my favorite actor, gave both my son and I what we often time couldn't seem to give each other. Some comfort and peace, and even sometimes, a reason to smile.

If you don't or have never had a pet, I don't expect you to understand. Just believe me when I say that having her here, kept both of us going sometimes. She broke up the monotony of going to radiation treatment and then coming home and just laying on the sofa doing nothing. I didn't have much energy to do anything.

And for Josh, I think she may have given him an outlet to chill and have fun for a while in a house that felt like a tomb at times.

The things I used to enjoy, I couldn't do anymore. I had no interest in them.

And even though I really loved my son, I just didn't have the strength, energy and sometimes, though I hate to admit, the right frame of mind to deal with him. So if you lose interest in things you used to love to do, all I'm saying is try to find something to replace that. I think it's important, it really helped me.

I'm not Superwomen?
When did that happen?

It was very important for me to drive myself to radiation. Someone had to be with me through the surgeries, but since I wasn't taking any drugs that kept me from driving, I had to drive to myself to radiation treatment. After my biopsy came back positive, my oldest sister changed her plans and stayed with me as long as she could. She and her family were moving to another country, but she didn't leave right away. She and my other sister were with me as much as they could be. They researched the internet and brought so many books that I could have opened a library. They read and talked and we hung out until they had to return to their homes and take care of their families. I let them do all of the reading because I didn't want to tell them that

I couldn't concentrate very well anymore. I used to have a book in every room of the house, but now I couldn't remember what I read so I just stopped reading.

My concession was to call the American Cancer Society. After I refused their help finding a support group, they sent me literature. I didn't read any of the books my sisters brought, but I did read some of the information the ACS sent to me. Didn't understand a whole lot, but I read some of it.

The time my sisters and I spent together meant so much to me. I loved to have them here. But it was extremely hard for me to accept that I had to have someone with me at times. Even harder that I couldn't do it all by myself.

We're a military family. Used to being apart and just making phone calls and writing letters. Going months, sometimes years without seeing each other. We grew up learning to rely only on ourselves. Mom taught us that women needed to be independent and able to care for themselves with or without a man around. And trust me, I took that to heart and tried to live my life without any help from others. Still don't like asking for help.

My sisters bent over backwards to be with me as much as they could. We were sisters by blood, but during this time, we became something more important, friends. Our relationships have changed because of my illness. It brought us a closeness that we never had before and remains to this day.

My oldest sister had to move to Korea before the partial mastectomy, she's back in the states now thank God, and my middle sister lives in North Georgia. As sick as she was my middle sister, Robin, was here as much as she could be. And being sick herself, it was no easy thing to do. I used to try to talk her out of coming because I worried about her so much. Sometimes she would just show up because she knew that if she called to tell me she was coming, I would try to convince her not to. It was a three hour drive on a good day. But she was here for all of the surgeries. And sometimes just to spend some time with me.

Without her here I think, actually, I know that I would have left the bandages on until they fell off naturally or became a petrified part of my body after the partial mastectomy. I could not stand the idea that part of me was gone. I was so afraid of what it would look like. To me my breasts were my greatest asset, my hair a close second. My reaction to what I saw was so bizarre. I saw what was not, if that makes sense. It was an awful sight, but it was ten times worse in my mind. Half of my breast was gone. Of course that wasn't true, but it's what I saw. After I stopped screaming and crying, when Robin finally convinced me to look again, it was not what I expected. A huge piece of my breast was gone, but I first saw most of my breast gone. And I know I wasn't in my right mind because I let her take a picture of it. She wanted to prove to me that I was still beautiful, so she sent it to someone we love, a man, and he came back and said that it was not so bad and that I was still beautiful. That did help me feel better.

When I finally realized what she had done, I was so embarrassed. But at the time, that reassurance from someone of the opposite sex, made me think that I just might be okay.

I think it's important to have someone with you when you take the bandages off. And if I was married, I'm telling you now, I know for sure it wouldn't be my husband. Unless there doctors', most men cannot handle seeing that kind of thing. I've always said that if men had to have the first baby, we wouldn't have so many children in this world.

Don't get me wrong, I love my men. Most, to me, are just not equipped to handle some situations. My brothers called very seldom through my illness, and NEVER came to see me. My dad didn't even want to talk about it. To him it was as if it never happened. And the male friend that meant so much to me also never came to see me during that time, and he lived less than five miles.

I equate what I went through in some ways to post partum depression. At the time it's the lowest of the low, but only you can come out of the funk that you're in. With or without help, you have to make it yourself. I'll say again, no one, whether they've been through it or not, can understand how you feel or what you're going through. It's impossible because, they are not you. You're going to expect them to understand. FORGET IT! Not gonna happen.

Do the support group things if you think it will work for you. Go and talk and cry about how you're life has changed. It has changed. I guess the group thing really does help some people. Me, I chose not to go that route. I'm not one for baring my soul to a bunch of strangers. I would have loved to be able to talk one on one, but that was not an option. The military didn't see the need for it. So, I was forced to go to depression classes, but I didn't tell them how I really felt. I said just enough for them to think I was okay. I've had a chance to see my medical records. They called me slightly depressed. Ya think!

Like I said, I did not bare my soul to strangers. I considered it a sign of weakness. I still don't open up about everything. Shoot, up until this happened I used to pride myself on only crying three times a year. Don't look at me the wrong way now, or the waterworks will start. But back then, I had to have control and not show weakness in any way, shape, or form. My sisters have found a way to break me from some of that. Doggone edumacated women!

Mama always said "God don't give you more than you can handle." Okay, so why did he choose me to "handle" this? Though I didn't pray like I should have, nor go to church, I did believe that whatever I was going through, someone else was going through worse. And I also felt, that this was happening to me for a reason. Don't know what that was, but there had to be one. This couldn't just be some random act. I could not accept that.

I did the "why me" thing pity parties, but only when I was alone. In front of others, the wall was up. I got very upset with myself when I was too sick to drive to radiation treatment one day. I had a song that I found on one of my cd's. If I started that song by the artist "Maxwell" as I was leaving, it would end just as I pulled up to the doctors' office for treatment. One day, I had to call a friend to drive me. It was devastating to me, because I had to rely on someone else. I think that he was genuinely happy to be able to do something for me. But to me, I was losing my independence. I was not in control. Even when my sister was here, I would drive us. Had to. Plus, I wanted her to think that I was doing alright.

I believe things like that helped me make it. Driving, listening to that one special song. Fighting to keep control of what I could. Not physically fighting, mentally trying to find a way to keep my edge. I do believe that because I made myself do those things, I kept myself strong. It kept me going.

Find something that's special to you. It's there. Make something your own, something good for your spirit. Even when you're feeling your worst, let that special something bring you back up.

And when the day comes, if it ever does, that you have to rely on someone else to help you. Let them do it. Most of the time they were just waiting for you to ask.

Being the type of person that I am, I still struggle with accepting help from others. But I have found that when

I ask, they are truly happy to do it. So, while you're sick, try to learn to rely on people when you need to.

Now, I'm not in any way saying, just stop doing for you. That would be the wrong thing to do. I'm just saying, let them in. You will be able to tell if they really want to help out or not. And if they don't, just remember not to ask them again.

Let them negative people go, but keep the ones that count

Before they found the cancer, I was so sick that I would sometimes pass out driving to work or have to hold on to walls in order to keep from falling over as I walked. If I got up from sitting to fast, I'd have to sit back down until the dizziness passed. Now those are times I prayed.

Remember that I was sick for a year and half before they found the cancer. People at work thought that I was faking being sick. Even the first primary care doctor told me that I needed to stop thinking that I was sick.

My blood tests came back abnormal several times, but nothing was done to try to figure out why I was weak, nauseous, dizzy, blacking out. Couldn't eat or sleep, but I was gaining weight. My hair was falling out.

Folks at work told me I had a bad attitude. DAH. I was still working full days, still doing my job. Being given more and more to do. And constantly being degraded and maligned because I wasn't always smiling and talking about my personal business all of the time. If I told them I didn't feel good, they would say things like "you're always sick." The difference was that while I was sick, I was still at work. Meeting deadlines and suspense's, help anyone that needed help if I could. Watching others being given awards and time off for work that someone else did, or staying home with sick kids without taking leave time. One of my bosses even told me that they wanted me at work so that they could keep eye on me and make sure I was okay. Think I believe that? Not! You better believe that if I or my child was ill, I better have a doctor's note or be at work. Sometimes I had to leave him home alone, sick, because he was a teenager.

I was just trying to make it through the work day so that I could go home to my child and try to be Mom for a few hours before collapsing. I was just barely surviving.

You know how some people say, cut the negative from your life. Well, I couldn't do that because I worked with it. What did I do? I had a few friends at work, one that I love dearly to this day. But some of the others, I cut them off. If it wasn't work related, I did not talk to them. Period. That's where I guess the "bad attitude" impression came in. I could have cared less; I felt that their attitudes were detrimental to my health and well being. I was truly sick enough without having to deal with that proverbial "knife in my back." And if I really didn't want to deal, I took what I called a "mental health day." It meant I had to take a day of personal leave, but it was worth it to not have to go in and "fake the funk" with people that I knew could care less about me or what I was and would have to go through.

I feel that I failed miserably at the Mom thing. I didn't realize that my child was suffering as much as I was. He was scared of losing the only parent he had. At the time, I didn't see that. So when he did things to rebel, I became mean. The more he rebelled the meaner I got. It was a vicious cycle that was killing us both. I so regret that my illness and stress caused us to fall apart. He had to grow up to fast and didn't have the chance to be a normal teenager. How hard that must have been. So easy to see now but not at the time.

It took years for me to realize what my illness had done to him. This illness, and then this cancer happened at a time when his best friend, my nephew Terry had to leave. So, he had some friends, but the only family he had besides me, was gone.

I apologized to him for the hateful mean things that I said and did. Thankfully, he has forgiven me, which in time allowed me to forgive myself.

My oldest sister and her husband actually took him to live with them for his senior year of high school. I was done with the cancer treatments by then, but still fighting a lot of the symptoms I had prior. And our relationship was so damaged that I didn't think it could ever be okay.

What happens to you affects everyone in your house. Everyone in your life. As hard as it is, you have to try to find a way to help them. Not to understand what's going on with you, but to understand that you are different. That life is different. For me, when the cancer treatments were finished, it was a chance for me to begin a new life. And try to do it better this time around.

How many of us get another chance?

Its okay to feel how you feel

Six years cancer free! A year after the DCIS, I had a cyst removed from my other breast, notice I'm not saying left or right, keep them guessing, that ended up being squaemous cell carcinoma, a form of skin cancer. In a place that never saw the sun mind you. It was the first time that any cyst was sent off for a pathology report. I still have problems with cysts and will forever.

And my symptoms prior to finding the cancer did not get better; they actually continued and got worse.

So was it Cancer Related Fatigue? I believe that some of it was, but I also knew that wasn't all that was wrong.

It took over a year of fighting after my final treatment for me to be allowed to have breast surgery. Reconstructive surgery was being considered a cosmetic procedure, which wasn't permitted at the time. Finally, I was allowed to have a breast reduction so that at least my babies would be the same size. I was never allowed to have the breast reconstructed to look close to normal. But I've learned to deal with the way I look on the outside, because my insides have healed. Now, that I am retired, I know that even if allowed I could not afford to have the plastic surgery to make my breast look okay. Even with insurance, I couldn't afford the co-pay for an overnight hospital stay or the operation.

Both of my eyes have been affected. At times, very painful! I actually lost most of the vision in my left eye for a period of time. A wonderful retina specialist resolved that and my sight returned, but the infection is incurable. And no one knows what causes the flair ups. I will have to use steroid drops off and on for the rest of my life, and drops for the pain when the infection flairs up. Or at least until someone finds a cure for this disease. Another reason not to cry, it really makes my eyes hurt.

I went to a baseball game with my sister, and passed out cold before the third inning. I had passed out by myself before, while driving or even just sitting in the house not feeling well. But never in front of other people like that. I somehow managed to get out of the public eye if I was feeling myself go down.

I have difficulty driving long distances. I call them "episodes." I have actually zoned out, driving miles without realizing I was not aware of what I was doing.

I suffer from degenerative disc disease and arthritis in my lower spine. I often wear a back brace when the pain becomes too hard to bare and the numbness in my legs has lasted more than a day or two. I also have arthritis in one hand and knee.

I had an operation on one of my toes that became so infected my toe literally exploded. I called and went to the doctors several times prior to that happening. Their solution was to keep wearing a surgical shoe or slipper, instead of combat boots. After that incident, there was no way to ignore that I had a problem. It was then that the doctors decided, yes, there really was something else wrong.

By the time I was allowed to see a specialist, I was literally wishing for death. And according to the medicine I know have to take, I was in pretty bad shape. The mental and physical abuse that I was taking on a daily basis, had become just too much. I wanted to be done and away from all of the things that I felt were killing me.

Very rarely do I eat a full meal. I can go days surviving on power drinks and water, because even the thought of food can make me nauseous.

And guess what? I suffer from migraine headaches. I am missing an artery or vein, something that carries blood to my head, on one side of my neck. How about that!

So, I'm being treated for who knows what. They never really figured it out before I retired; I think they were just glad to see me go. And I was oh so happy to be gone.

I've fought the doctors, my superiors, and others who didn't believe what I was saying. Someone in my organization even had the nerve to say that I should be grateful for whatever they gave me because of my attitude.

I've been through some traumatic experiences in my life.

My son, having life threatening surgery when he was only six months old.

Holding my mothers' hand and watching her breath her last breath.

Three years after her death I found my Dad dead in his apartment.

As hard as these experiences were for me to deal with, nothing changed my life more than the ordeal of breast cancer.

I feel like a part of me died the day that the surgeon walked through that door with the news. And I believe that a part of me did, but I was re-born as a different person. Determined to fight, and what a fight it was, and still is.

It's not over yet!

I was back at work the next business day after my last radiation treatment. I walked in there, some people spoke, some acted like I had the plague. But I was there.

The problem with that was, not only was I still sick, but I still had doctors' appointments and more treatment to go through.

Don't be surprised if people think that once you're done with surgeries and radiation, your okay. That was the perception I got. I think a lot of times; it's easier for them to deal with if they try to deny the fact that you had anything wrong in the first place. Especially something like cancer.

As I said before, my cancer ended up being estrogen receptive, which meant that I couldn't take any kind of hormone replacement therapy and we had to be careful which of the treatment drugs I took after that. My oncologist worked with me very closely to make sure that I reacted well to the drugs.

I also had to have procrit and vitamin shots every few weeks, because my blood tests were still abnormal. So I spent a lot of time at different doctors' office. It became an issue with some of the people I worked with. Some of them were upset because to them I was out of work to much. Mind you, I tried to make my appointments as early or as late as possible, so that I wouldn't be gone too long. I even spent many lunch times at the doctors' office, so that I didn't have to miss any work time. Many times I would also work through my lunch hour so that I could make up lost work time. I was always early and often stayed late, but that still didn't matter. I was actually told that coming in early didn't count because no one else was there to prove that I was. But I still did it so that I could have my fifteen or thirty minutes of peace before the rest of them came in.

Still had the problem with cysts. It was actually during the after cancer treatment that my oncologist requested one of the cysts be removed and biopsied. That's when we found out that I had skin cancer. Oh joy, another huge scar to deal with.

So there is still a lot to go through once you're "cured."

In retrospect maybe I would have received better treatment at work if I had told them all of this. I don't really think so. It was as if I had leprosy and not breast cancer.

Try it though.

Maybe if you tell them that you are not considered cancer free until you have no reoccurrences for five years.

Maybe if you tell them that you still have to be checked by your oncologist monthly to be sure the meds are working the way they should.

That your primary doctor will want to check occasionally to be sure you're healing without complications.

That it still hurts sometimes when you take a shower or get dressed, or someone brushes up against you by accident.

That you still get tired easily because your entire immune system has been compromised.

Just maybe, they will try to understand.

I still had some issues going on with my body. A lot of the things that were going on prior to the breast cancer were still going on. And continue to this day. So my battle is not over, now, it's just a battle that I can deal with without the mental torment of having to deal with people who could care less about you.

Believe it or not, I have less really bad days now. I have the time to take better care of myself and limit the amount of stress in my life.

And when I feel myself going down, I have the time to try doing something about it.

So if you can change your situation, please try to do it. What a difference it will make.

IN YOUR OWN UNIQUENESS, YOU CAN FIND YOURSELF!

All of the feelings I went through didn't happen all at once. Or maybe they did start on the day the doctor told me I had cancer. I just know that, sometimes I felt guilty or lonely, or depressed all at once. Every day was a mixture of emotions and feelings. And like I said a serious roller coaster ride. I hate roller coasters.

Then one day I woke up and realized that I truly had survived breast cancer. I was a survivor. WOW! No more. I was okay.

I don't know about you, but every once in a while my breast still hurts. At first I used to think, oh my goodness, here I go again. But now I realize that it's going to hurt sometimes. Actually they both do. And it's probably something that happened before the cancer I just didn't remember it. So now I just consider these aches and pain a part of life.

For months after I was told that I was cancer free, I still worried that it would happen again. Sometimes, even now, I get anxious about it.

But it doesn't consume me. It's not part of my everyday life anymore.

I truly believe that surviving breast cancer is one of the hardest things you can do. This disease, cancer, in any form or stage ravages your body and mind. It seems to take away your independence, your hopes and dreams, life as you know it. At least for a while. But for me, losing a part of myself that was visible to everyone was one of the hardest things I have ever gone through.

And, having to make all of the decisions was over whelming to me at times.

Do I have the surgery the doctor is suggesting?

Do I let them take a little, or do I try to fight to have my entire breast removed so that I don't have to go through this again? Sometimes, you do have that choice. I didn't.

Do I really want to go through the radiation and or chemotherapy that they say "may" save my life?

No one can decide what is best for you. They can recommend and give opinions, but the ultimate choice is up to you.

Not having the know how to deal with the physical effects it had on my body, really threw me for a loop sometimes. What seemed to work one day to help me feel better, didn't always work the next. That was especially true when it came to food. There are foods even now, that I used to eat but can't anymore. Now, on the flip side, I can eat some things that I considered extremely gross before.

I learned by a lot by trial and error some of the products, clothes, foods that would give me comfort and ease some of the side effects. And it was and I am pretty sure will be different for each and every one of you that have to go through this. You have to take the time to find out what works for you. I hope that some of the things I've shared might help.

I had to learn how to be selfish sometimes when it came to myself, something that was also very hard for me. Selfish without forgetting that your life involves other people too. And you have to think about what this is doing to them.

Through it all I found out that if you don't take care of yourself, you have no one to blame but yourself.

You have to learn to find doctors that give a damn. Sorry, I cannot find any other way to say that. If you don't do this, in my opinion, you will suffer more than you need to.

Try to learn to live one day at a time. Another old cliché, but to me it seems so true.

I stopped making plans, because that day would come and I might not feel like going out to meet someone, or go shopping, or doing whatever. So instead of trying to go out and do things because I told someone I would, I just didn't make plans.

The only thing I did consistently was keep my doctor appointments. Not really too much choice on that. Actually you do have a choice, but don't make a decision you may later regret.

Sure there were plenty of times that I didn't want to go. That I wanted to give up and just let this disease and how I felt defeat me. But I didn't give up or give in. And please don't you either.

Even now, years later, I don't want to go get my breasts squished by that man made machine. But I do, because I know what the consequences could be if I don't. I am a firm advocate of those fifteen minutes of pain and torture, because it saved my life. I used to avoid it like the plague, but if you talk to me now, I'm probably going to ask you sooner or later if you've had a physical. And, to me that means you also had a mammogram.

Because to me it's not a complete physical unless you have.

My point is, when you have survived the mental and physical anguish of what cancer does to your body and mind, and the ignorance of some of the folks around you. YOU ARE A SURVIVOR. No one can ever take that away from you.

So, cut that hair, slap on that grease, scream, cry, and find a way to smile, cut the negative out of your life, keep the good, just find a way to endure, because you are worth it. And however, you feel while you're going through this. It's OK!